Asia

For

Diabetics

Thai, Chinese, Vietnamese & Japanese
diabetes friendly recipes

Table Of Contents

Table Of Contents

Terms Of Use Agreement

   Disclaimer

Kung Pao Chicken

Cashew Chicken

Beef and Broccoli

Shrimp Fried Rice

Sweet-and-Sour Pork

Light 'n' Crispy Egg Rolls

Asian Flank Steak

Thai-Style Veggie Pizza

Asian Turkey Steaks

Caesar Salad with Tofu Croutons

Asian Vegetable Lo Mein

Thai Spinach Dip

Asparagus and Carrots with Asian Vinaigrette

Baked Vegetable Tempura

Crispy Tofu and Vegetables

Ginger Chicken with Rice Noodles

Sesame-Ginger Turkey Wraps

Beef Satay with Peanut Sauce

Ginger Pork with Tofu

Terms Of Use Agreement

Copyright 2015
All Rights Reserved

The author hereby asserts his/her right to be identified as the author of this work in accordance with sections 77 to 78 of the copyright, design and patents act 1988 as well as all other applicable international, federal, state and local laws.

Without limiting the rights under copyright reserved above, no part of this book may be reproduced, stored in or introduced into retrieval system, or transmitted, in any form or by any electronic or mechanical means, without the prior written permission of the copyright owner of this book, except by a reviewer who may quote brief passages.

There are no resale rights included. Anyone re - selling, or using this material in any way other than what is outlined within this book will be prosecuted to the full extend of the law.

Every effort had been made to fulfill requirements with regard to reproducing copyrighted material. The author and the publisher will be glad to certify any omissions at the earliest opportunity.

Disclaimer

The author and the publisher have used their best efforts in preparing this book. The author and the publisher make no representation or warranties with respect to the accuracy, fitness, applicability, or completeness of the contents of this work and specifically disclaim all warranties, including without limitation warranties of fitness for a particular purpose. This work is sold with the understanding that author and the publisher is not engaged in rendering legal, or any other professional services.

The information contained in this book is strictly for educational purposes. Therefore, if you wish to apply ideas contained within this book, you are taking full responsibility for your actions. The author and the publisher disclaim any warranties (express or implied), merchantability, or fitness for any particular purpose. The Author and The publisher shall in no event be held responsible / liable to any party for any indirect, direct, special, punitive, incidental, or other consequential damages arising directly or indirectly from any use of this material, which is provided 'as is', and without warranties.

The author and the publisher do not warrant the performance, applicability, or effectiveness of any websites and other medias listed or linked to in this publication. All links are for informative purposes only and are not warranted for contents, accuracy, or any other implied or explicit purpose.

Kung Pao Chicken

Ingredients:

- 5 teaspoons reduced-sodium soy sauce
- 2 teaspoons dry sherry
- 2 teaspoons toasted sesame oil
- 10 ounces skinless, boneless chicken breast halves, cut into 1/2-inch pieces
- 3 tablespoons water
- 2 tablespoons rice vinegar
- 1 tablespoon granulated sugar or granulated sugar substitute or brown sugar substitute* equivalent to 1 tablespoon sugar
- 1 teaspoon cornstarch
- 4 teaspoons canola oil
- 4 dried red chili peppers, seeded and broken into small pieces
- 4 green onions, cut into 1-inch piece
- 2 cups coarsely chopped bok choy
- 2 teaspoons grated fresh ginger
- 1 1/3 cups hot cooked brown rice
- 1/4 cup chopped unsalted dry roasted peanuts

Methods:

- In a medium bowl stir together 2 teaspoons of the soy sauce, the sherry, and sesame oil; add chicken and toss to coat.
- Marinate at room temperature for 20 minutes. Meanwhile, for sauce:
- Stir together the remaining 3 teaspoons soy sauce, the water, rice vinegar, sugar, and cornstarch; set aside.
- In a large skillet heat 2 teaspoons of the canola oil over medium-high heat. Add marinated chicken; stir-fry until nearly cooked through. Remove chicken.
- Add the remaining 2 teaspoons oil. Add chili peppers and green onions; stir-fry for 1 minute. Add bok choy and ginger; stir-fry for 1 minute more. Add the sauce; cook until bubbly. Serve with hot cooked rice. Sprinkle with peanuts.

Cashew Chicken

Ingredients:

- 2 tablespoons reduced-sodium soy sauce
- 1 tablespoon cornstarch
- 2 teaspoons grated fresh ginger or 1/2 teaspoon ground ginger
- 2 teaspoons toasted sesame oil
- 12 ounces skinless, boneless chicken breast halves, cut into 1/2-inch pieces
- 2 tablespoons water
- 2 tablespoons oyster sauce
- 1 6 - ounce package frozen snow pea pods
- 1/3 cup unsalted dry roasted cashews, coarsely chopped
- 3 teaspoons canola oil
- 1 medium red onion, cut into thin wedges
- 1 medium red sweet pepper, seeded and cut into bite-size pieces
- 3 cloves garlic, minced
- 1 8 - ounce can sliced water chestnuts, drained

Methods:

- In a medium bowl stir together soy sauce, cornstarch, ginger, and sesame oil; add chicken and toss to coat.
- Cover and marinate at room temperature for 20 minutes.
- Meanwhile, for sauce: In a small bowl stir together the water and oyster sauce; set aside. Rinse pea pods under cold running water to thaw; set aside to drain well.
- Heat a large nonstick skillet or wok over medium-high heat. Add cashews to hot skillet; cook about 3 minutes or until nuts start to brown, stirring frequently.
- Remove from skillet; set aside. Add 1 teaspoon of the canola oil to skillet; add onion and stir-fry for 1 minute.
- Add sweet pepper, pea pods, and garlic; stir-fry for 1 minute. Stir in water chestnuts.
- Remove vegetables from skillet. Add the remaining 2 teaspoons canola oil to skillet; add chicken mixture and stir-fry for 2 to 3 minutes or until chicken is cooked through.

- Return vegetables to skillet.
- Add the sauce; heat through, scraping up any browned bits from bottom of skillet.
- Transfer to a serving dish or plates.
- Sprinkle with the roasted cashews.

Beef and Broccoli

Ingredients:

- 3 teaspoons cornstarch
- 1 tablespoon reduced-sodium soy sauce
- 3 cloves garlic, minced
- 1/4 teaspoon crushed red pepper
- 12 ounces boneless beef top sirloin steak, bias-sliced 1/8-inch thick*
- 4 ounces Chinese egg noodles or whole wheat vermicelli
- 1 pound fresh broccoli
- 3 tablespoons hoisin sauce
- 2 tablespoons water
- 2 teaspoons toasted sesame oil
- 1 tablespoon canola oil
- 3/4 cup reduced-sodium beef broth
- 1 cup quartered and/or halved cherry tomatoes

Methods:

- In a medium bowl stir together 2 teaspoons of the cornstarch, the soy sauce, garlic, and crushed red

- pepper; add beef and stir to coat. Marinate at room temperature for 20 minutes.
- Meanwhile, cook Chinese noodles or vermicelli according to package directions, except omit salt; drain and set aside.
- Cut broccoli into 2-inch florets. Peel broccoli stem and cut into 1/2-inch slices; set aside. For sauce: Stir together hoisin sauce, the water, sesame oil, and the remaining 1 teaspoon cornstarch; set aside.
- In a very large skillet or wok heat canola oil over medium-high heat. Add beef mixture; stir-fry for 1 to 2 minutes or until still slightly pink in center. Remove beef mixture; set aside.
- Stir beef broth into skillet, scraping up any browned bits from bottom of skillet. Add broccoli; bring to boiling.
- Reduce heat to medium. Cover and cook for 3 to 4 minutes or until broccoli is crisp-tender.
- Add sauce to broccoli; cook and stir until thickened.
- Add beef and tomatoes; heat through. Serve over cooked Chinese noodles or whole wheat vermicelli.

Shrimp Fried Rice

Ingredients:

- 12 ounces fresh or frozen medium shrimp in shells
- 1 egg
- 2 egg whites
- 4 teaspoons canola oil
- 1/2 cup chopped carrot (1 medium)
- 1/2 cup chopped celery (1 stalk)
- 1/2 cup sliced fresh mushrooms
- 1/2 cup sliced green onions (4)
- 1 teaspoon grated fresh ginger
- 2 cups unsalted cooked brown rice, chilled
- 1/2 14 - ounce can bean sprouts, rinsed

Methods:

- Thaw shrimp, if frozen. Peel and devein shrimp. Rinse shrimp; pat dry with paper towels and set aside.
- In a small bowl beat together egg and egg whites; set aside. In a large skillet or wok heat 2

teaspoons of the oil over medium-high heat. Add shrimp; stir-fry about 2 minutes or until shrimp are opaque.
- Remove shrimp; set aside.
- Add the remaining 2 teaspoons oil to the skillet or wok.
- Add carrot, celery, mushrooms, green onions, and ginger; stir-fry for 3 to 4 minutes or until vegetables are tender.
- Add egg mixture; let stand for 5 to 10 seconds or until egg sets on bottom but remains runny on top. Add rice and bean sprouts.
- Turn and toss mixture continuously for 1 minute. Stir in shrimp, peas, and soy sauce; heat through.

Sweet-and-Sour Pork

Ingredients:

- 1 large red sweet pepper, quartered and seeded
- 1 teaspoon water
- 1 8 - ounce can pineapple chunks
- 2 tablespoons reduced-sodium soy sauce
- Brown sugar substitute equivalent to 1 tablespoon brown sugar
- 1 tablespoon cornstarch
- 2 teaspoons grated fresh ginger
- 2 cloves garlic
- 2 teaspoons rice vinegar
- 4 teaspoons canola oil
- 1 medium green sweet pepper, seeded and cut into 1-inch pieces
- 1 8 - ounce can bamboo shoots

Methods:

- Place red sweet pepper quarters, cut sides down, in a microwave-safe dish. Add the water. Cover with plastic wrap.

- Microwave on 100 percent power (high) for 4 to 5 minutes or until tender. Let stand about 10 minutes or until skin easily peels from flesh; remove and discard skin.
- Place red sweet pepper in a food processor; cover and process until smooth.
- Drain pineapple chunks, reserving 1/3 cup of the juice; set pineapple chunks aside.
- Add the reserved 1/3 cup pineapple juice, the soy sauce, brown sugar, cornstarch, ginger, garlic, and rice vinegar to red sweet pepper in food processor. Cover and process until combined; set aside.
- In a large skillet heat 1 teaspoon of the oil over medium-high heat. Add green sweet pepper; stir-fry about 2 minutes or until crisp-tender.
- Add bamboo shoots; stir-fry for 30 seconds.
- Remove vegetables from skillet.
- Add the remaining 3 teaspoons oil to skillet.
- Add pork strips; stir-fry for 2 to 3 minutes or just until done. Add the red sweet pepper mixture; cook and stir about 30 seconds or until thickened and bubbly.

- Cook and stir for 2 minutes more. Stir in green sweet pepper mixture and pineapple chunks; heat through.
- Serve over napa cabbage.

Light 'n' Crispy Egg Rolls

Ingredients:

- Nonstick cooking spray
- 2 teaspoons toasted sesame oil or canola oil
- 8 ounces lean pork loin, cut into 1/2-inch pieces, or ground pork
- 1/2 cup chopped red sweet pepper
- 1 teaspoon grated fresh ginger or 1/4 teaspoon ground ginger
- 1 clove garlic, minced
- 3/4 cup finely chopped bok choy or Chinese (napa) cabbage
- 1/2 cup chopped canned water chestnuts
- 1/2 cup coarsely shredded carrot
- 1/4 cup sliced green onions
- 1/4 cup bottled light Asian sesame ginger vinaigrette
- 8 egg roll wrappers

Methods:

- Preheat oven to 450 degrees F. Lightly coat a large baking sheet with nonstick cooking spray; set aside.
- For filling: In a medium nonstick skillet, heat oil over medium-high heat.
- Add pork, sweet pepper, ginger, and garlic. Cook for 3 to 4 minutes or until pork is no longer pink, stirring occasionally.
- If using ground pork, drain off fat. Add bok choy, water chestnuts, carrot, and green onions to pork mixture in skillet.
- Cook and stir about 1 minute more or until any liquid evaporates. Stir in vinaigrette. Cool filling slightly.
- For each egg roll, place an egg roll wrapper on a flat surface with a corner pointing toward you. Spoon about 1/3 cup of the filling across and just below center of each egg roll wrapper.
- Fold bottom corner over filling, tucking it under on the other side.
- Fold side corners over filling, forming an envelope shape. Roll egg roll toward remaining corner.

Moisten top corner with water; press firmly to seal.
- Place egg rolls, seam sides down, on the prepared baking sheet.
- Coat the tops and sides of the egg rolls with nonstick cooking spray.
- Bake for 15 to 18 minutes or until egg rolls are golden brown and crisp.
- Cool slightly before serving.

Asian Flank Steak

Ingredients:

- 1 1 1/4 - pound beef flank steak
- 1/2 cup beef broth
- 1/3 cup bottled hoisin sauce
- 1/4 cup reduced-sodium soy sauce
- 1/4 cup sliced green onions
- 3 tablespoons dry sherry or apple or orange juice
- 1 teaspoon grated fresh ginger
- 4 cloves garlic, minced

Methods:

- Trim fat from steak. Place steak in a resealable plastic bag set in a shallow dish.
- Combine broth, hoisin, soy sauce, onions, sherry, ginger, and garlic; pour over steak.
- Seal the bag; turn to coat.
- Marinate in the refrigerator for 4 to 24 hours, turning bag occasionally.
- Drain steak, discarding marinade. Grill on the rack of an uncovered grill directly over medium coals

for 17 to 21 minutes or to medium doneness (160 degree F), turning once.
- To serve, thinly slice steak across the grain. Makes 6 (2-1/2-ounce cooked meat) servings.

Thai-Style Veggie Pizza

Ingredients:

- 1 8 - inch Italian bread shell (such as Boboli brand)
- Nonstick cooking spray
- 1/2 cup sliced fresh shiitake or button mushrooms
- 1/3 cup fresh pea pods, cut into thin strips
- 2 tablespoons coarsely shredded carrot
- 2 tablespoons sliced green onion
- 2 -3 tablespoons bottled peanut sauce
- 1 tablespoon chopped peanuts
- Fresh cilantro leaves

Methods:

- Preheat oven to 450 degrees F.
- Place bread shell on an ungreased baking sheet.
- Bake for 5 to 7 minutes or until lightly browned and crisp.
- Meanwhile, lightly coat an unheated medium nonstick skillet with nonstick cooking spray. Preheat skillet over medium heat.

- Add mushrooms, pea pods, and carrot; cook about 2 minutes or just until tender. Stir in green onion.
- Remove from heat.
- Carefully spread hot bread shell with peanut sauce.
- Top with hot vegetable mixture; sprinkle with peanuts and cilantro leaves.
- Cut in half to serve.

Asian Turkey Steaks

Ingredients:

- 3/4 cup orange juice
- 2 teaspoons cornstarch
- 2 tablespoons reduced-sodium soy sauce
- 2 teaspoons grated fresh ginger
- 4 teaspoons hoisin sauce
- 1 pound turkey breast tenderloins, cut crosswise into 4 portions

Methods:

- Transfer 2 tablespoons of the orange juice to a small bowl. Stir in cornstarch; set aside.
- In a 4-quart pressure cooker, combine the remaining orange juice, the soy sauce, and ginger.
- Spread 1 teaspoon of the hoisin sauce on one side of each turkey portion. Place turkey portions, hoisin sides up, in pressure cooker. Lock lid in place.

- Over high heat, bring cooker up to 15 pounds pressure. Reduce heat just enough to maintain high pressure. Cook for 3 minutes. Remove cooker from heat. Allow pressure to decrease naturally.
- Carefully remove lid, tilting it away from you to allow steam to escape. Using a slotted spoon, transfer turkey to a cutting board; thinly slice turkey.
- Keep warm.
- For sauce: Strain cooking liquid. Return to pressure cooker.
- Stir orange juice-cornstarch mixture; add to liquid in cooker.
- Cook and stir until thickened and bubbly; cook and stir for 2 minutes more.
- Serve sauce over turkey.
- If desired, sprinkle with green onion and serve with brown rice.

Caesar Salad with Tofu Croutons

Ingredients:

- 2/3 cup firm cubed silken-style tofu
- 2 tablespoons lemon juice
- 1 tablespoon water
- 3 cloves garlic, halved
- 1 teaspoon Dijon-style mustard
- 1/8 teaspoon salt
- 1/8 teaspoon ground black pepper
- 1/4 cup soybean cooking oil
- 10 cups torn romaine
- 2 cups cut-up red, yellow, and/or orange cherry and/or pear tomatoes
- 1/4 cup pitted kalamata or ripe olives, cut up
- 1 Tofu Croutons
- 1/4 cup finely shredded Parmesan cheese

Methods:

- For dressing, in a food processor or blender, combine silken-style tofu, lemon juice, the water, garlic, mustard, salt, and pepper.
- Cover and process or blend until smooth, scraping down side as needed.
- With processor or blender running, slowly add the 1/4 cup cooking oil in a steady stream.
- If necessary, stir in additional water to thin dressing. Set aside.
- To serve, in a very large bowl, combine romaine, tomatoes, olives, and Tofu Croutons.
- Add dressing; toss gently to coat.
- Sprinkle with Parmesan cheese.

Asian Vegetable Lo Mein

Ingredients:

- 1 cup dried shiitake or Chinese black mushrooms (1 ounce)
- 1 cup boiling water
- 6 ounces dried noodles
- 2 egg whites
- 1 egg
- 2 teaspoons cooking oil
- 2 teaspoons toasted sesame oil
- 2 teaspoons finely chopped fresh ginger
- 1/2 teaspoon crushed red pepper
- 3 cloves garlic, minced
- 2 cups sugar snap peas or pea pods, halved
- 1 red sweet pepper, cut into thin bite-size strips
- 1/4 cup light teriyaki sauce

Methods:

- In a small bowl combine mushrooms and the 1 cup boiling water. Cover and let stand for 20 minutes.

- Drain mushrooms, reserving 1/2 cup liquid. Chop mushrooms and set aside.
- Meanwhile, in a large saucepan cook noodles in additional boiling water for 5 minutes; drain.
- Return noodles to saucepan; cover and keep warm.
- For egg strips, combine egg whites and whole egg.
- In a 10-inch nonstick skillet heat 1 teaspoon of the cooking oil and 1 teaspoon of the sesame oil over medium heat.
- Pour egg mixture into skillet. Lift and tilt the skillet to form a thin layer of egg on the bottom. Cook, without stirring, for 2 to 3 minutes or just until set. Slide out onto a cutting board; cool slightly. Cut into 2x1/2-inch strips; set aside.
- In the same skillet heat the remaining 1 teaspoon cooking oil and the remaining 1 teaspoon sesame oil over medium-high heat.
- Add mushrooms, ginger, crushed red pepper , and garlic.
- Cook and stir for 1 minute.
- Add snap peas and sweet pepper; cook and stir for 2 minutes more. Add the reserved mushroom

liquid and the teriyaki sauce. Bring to boiling. Boil gently, uncovered, for 3 minutes.
- Add the egg strips and vegetable mixture to cooked noodles; toss gently to combine.
- Serve immediately.

Thai Spinach Dip

Ingredients:

- 1 cup chopped fresh spinach
- 1 8 - ounce carton light dairy sour cream
- 1 8 - ounce carton plain low-fat yogurt
- 1/4 cup snipped fresh mint
- 1/4 cup finely chopped peanuts
- 1/4 cup peanut butter
- 1 tablespoon honey
- 1 tablespoon reduced-sodium soy sauce
- 1 -2 teaspoons crushed red pepper

Methods:

- In a medium bowl, combine spinach, sour cream, and yogurt.
- Stir in the snipped mint, the 1/4 cup chopped peanuts, the peanut butter, honey, soy sauce, and crushed red pepper.
- Cover and chill for at least 2 hours. If desired, garnish with additional chopped peanuts and fresh mint leaves.

- Serve with vegetable dippers.
- Enjoy!

Asparagus and Carrots with Asian Vinaigrette

Ingredients:

- 8 ounces baby carrots with tops, trimmed to 2 inches, or packaged peeled baby carrots
- 12 asparagus spears
- 4 cups torn red-tip leaf lettuce or leaf lettuce
- 1 cup fresh enoki mushrooms
- 1 recipe Asian Vinaigrette
- 2 teaspoons sesame seeds, toasted (optional)

Methods:

- In a medium skillet cook carrots, covered, in a small amount of boiling water for 2 minutes.
- Meanwhile, snap off and discard woody bases from asparagus.
- If desired, scrape off scales from asparagus spears.
- Add asparagus spears to carrots.
- Cover and cook for 4 to 6 minutes more or until vegetables are crisp-tender.

- Drain; immediately plunge vegetables into ice water. Let stand for 1 minute. Drain and pat dry.
- Line salad plates with lettuce.
- Arrange carrots, asparagus, and mushrooms on lettuce.
- Drizzle with Asian Vinaigrette.
- Sprinkle with sesame seeds.

Baked Vegetable Tempura

Ingredients:

- Nonstick cooking spray
- 1 1/2 cups panko crumbs (Japanese-style bread crumbs)
- 1/4 teaspoon salt
- 1 1/2 cups cauliflower flowerets
- 1 1/2 cups small fresh mushrooms, stems removed
- 1 medium sweet potato, peeled and cut into 3 1/2-inch strips
- 1 small zucchini, sliced 1/4 inch thick
- 1 small red onion, sliced 1/2 inch thick and separated into rings
- 1 cup green beans
- 1 cup sugar snap peas
- 1/4 cup all-purpose flour
- 2 slightly beaten eggs
- 2 tablespoons margarine or butter, melted
- 1 recipe Honey-Mustard Sauce

Methods:

- Coat a 15 x 10 x 1-inch baking pan with cooking spray; set aside.
- In a medium bowl combine panko crumbs and salt.
- In a large bowl toss the vegetables in flour, shaking to remove any excess flour.
- Dip the vegetables, a few at a time, into the eggs, then into the panko crumb mixture to coat.
- Place the vegetables in a single layer in the prepared baking pan.
- Drizzle the vegetables with melted margarine.
- Bake, uncovered, in a 450 degrees degree oven for 9 to 11 minutes or until vegetables are golden brown, gently stirring twice.
- Serve immediately with Honey-Mustard Sauce.

Crispy Tofu and Vegetables

Ingredients:

- 1 10 1/2 - 12.3 - ounce package light extra-firm tofu (fresh bean curd), drained
- 3 tablespoons reduced-sodium soy sauce
- 8 green onions
- 8 ounces snow pea pods (2 cups), strings and tips removed
- 1 tablespoon toasted sesame oil
- 1 teaspoon grated fresh ginger or 1/2 teaspoon ground ginger
- 1 clove garlic, minced
- 1 red sweet pepper, seeded and cut into long, thin strips
- 1 yellow sweet pepper, seeded and cut into long, thin strips
- 3 tablespoons cornmeal

Methods:

- Cut tofu crosswise into eight slices.

- Arrange slices in one layer on a large plate or jelly-roll pan.
- Pour soy sauce over tofu; turn slices to coat and let stand for 1 hour.
- Meanwhile, cut root ends off green onions.
- Cut off dark green portion of onions, leaving 3 inches of white and light green.
- Cut green onions in half lengthwise, forming 16 long strips.
- Set aside.
- Cut pea pods in half lengthwise. Set aside.
- Pour oil into a large nonstick skillet. Preheat over medium-high heat.
- Stir-fry fresh ginger and garlic for 30 seconds.
- Add sweet pepper strips and stir-fry for 1 minute. Add green onions and pea pods; stir-fry for 2 to 3 minutes more or until crisp-tender.
- Drain tofu, reserving soy sauce.
- Stir reserved soy sauce and ground ginger into cooked vegetables; transfer vegetable mixture to a serving platter.
- Cover and keep warm.
- Carefully dip tofu slices in cornmeal to lightly coat both sides.

- Cook in same skillet for 3 minutes on each side or until crisp and hot, using a spatula to turn carefully.
- Serve tofu slices with vegetables.
- Sprinkle with sesame seeds.

Ginger Chicken with Rice Noodles

Ingredients:

- 2 tablespoons very finely chopped green onion
- 1 1/2 teaspoons grated fresh ginger
- 3 cloves garlic, minced
- 1 teaspoon olive oil
- 1/8 teaspoon salt
- 2 skinless, boneless chicken breast halves
- 2 ounces dried rice noodles
- 1/2 cup chopped carrot
- 1/2 teaspoon finely shredded lime peel
- 1 tablespoon lime juice
- 2 teaspoons olive oil
- 2 tablespoons coarsely chopped peanuts
- 1 -2 tablespoons snipped fresh cilantro

Methods:

- For rub, in a small bowl, combine green onion, ginger, garlic, the 1 teaspoon oil, and the salt.

- Sprinkle evenly over chicken; rub in with your fingers.
- Place chicken on the rack of an uncovered grill directly over medium coals.
- Grill for 12 to 15 minutes or until tender and no longer pink (170 degree F), turning once.
- Thinly slice chicken diagonally; set aside.
- Meanwhile, in a large saucepan, cook rice noodles and carrot in a large amount of boiling water for 3 to 4 minutes or just until noodles are tender; drain.
- Rinse with cold water; drain again. Use kitchen scissors to snip noodles into short lengths.
- In a medium bowl, stir together lime peel, lime juice, and the 2 teaspoons oil. Add noodle mixture and cilantro; toss gently to coat.
- Divide noodle mixture between two individual bowls; arrange chicken slices on noodle mixture.
- Sprinkle with peanuts and serve.

Sesame-Ginger Turkey Wraps

Ingredients:

- Nonstick cooking spray
- 3 turkey thighs, skinned (3-1/2 to 4 pounds)
- 1 cup bottled sesame-ginger stir-fry sauce
- 1/4 cup water
- 1 16 - ounce package shredded broccoli
- 12 8 - inches flour tortillas, warmed
- 3/4 cup sliced green onions

Methods:

- Lightly coat the inside of a slow cooker with nonstick cooking spray.
- Place turkey thighs in prepared cooker. In a small bowl stir together stir-fry sauce and water. Pour over turkey in cooker.
- Cover and cook on low-heat setting for 6 to 7 hours or on high-heat setting for 3 to 3-1/2 hours.
- Remove turkey from slow cooker; cool slightly. Remove turkey from bones; discard bones.

- Using two forks, shred turkey into bite-size pieces.
- Place broccoli slaw mix in sauce mixture in slow cooker. Stir to coat; cover and let stand for 5 minutes.
- Remove from cooker with a slotted spoon.
- To assemble, place some of the turkey on each warmed tortilla.
- Top with some of the broccoli mixture and green onions.
- Spoon some of the sauce from cooker on top of onions.
- Roll up and serve immediately.

Beef Satay with Peanut Sauce

Ingredients:

- 1 1 - 1 1/4 - pound beef flank steak
- 1/3 cup light teriyaki sauce
- 1/2 teaspoon bottled hot pepper sauce
- 1 medium green or red sweet pepper, cut into 3/4-inch pieces
- 4 green onions, cut into 1-inch pieces
- 3 tablespoons reduced-fat or regular peanut butter
- 3 tablespoons water
- 2 tablespoons light teriyaki sauce

Methods:

- Trim fat from meat. Thinly slice meat across grain into bite-size strips.
- For marinade: In medium bowl, combine 1/3 cup teriyaki sauce and 1/4 teaspoon of the hot pepper sauce.
- Add meat; toss gently to coat.

- Cover and marinate in the refrigerator for 30 minutes. If using wooden skewers, soak in water for 30 minutes before using.
- Drain meat, reserving marinade.
- On wooden or metal skewers, thread meat, accordion-style, alternating with sweet pepper and green onion.
- Brush with marinade.
- Grill kabobs on rack of uncovered grill directly over medium coals for 3 to 4 minutes or until meat is slightly pink in center, turning once halfway through grilling.
- For peanut sauce: In small saucepan, combine peanut butter, the water, 2 tablespoons teriyaki sauce, and remaining hot pepper sauce.
- Cook and stir over medium heat just until smooth and heated through.
- Serve kabobs with peanut sauce.

Ginger Pork with Tofu

Ingredients:

- 1 ounce dried shiitake mushrooms
- Boiling water
- 3 tablespoons reduced-sodium soy sauce
- 1 tablespoon cornstarch
- 1 tablespoon rice vinegar
- Nonstick cooking spray
- 8 ounces lean boneless pork, cut into thin bite-size strips
- 2 tablespoons grated fresh ginger
- 1 large clove garlic, minced
- 1/8 teaspoon cayenne pepper
- 1/2 cup sliced green onions
- 1 14 - 16 - ounce package extra-firm tub-style tofu (fresh bean curd), cut into 1-inch cubes
- 2 cups fresh pea pods, strings and tips removed
- 1 teaspoon toasted sesame oil
- 2 cups hot cooked brown rice (optional)
- 2 teaspoons sesame seeds, toasted (optional)

Methods:

- Place dried mushrooms in a medium bowl; add enough boiling water to cover. Let stand for 30 minutes.
- Drain, reserving 1 cup of the soaking liquid. Strain the reserved soaking liquid.
- Cut off tough stems of mushrooms and discard. Slice mushroom caps; set aside.
- In a small bowl, combine reserved soaking liquid, soy sauce, cornstarch, and rice vinegar; stir well to dissolve cornstarch.
- Lightly coat an unheated wok or large skillet with nonstick cooking spray.
- Preheat skillet over medium-high heat.
- Cook pork in hot skillet for 2 to 3 minutes or until no longer pink.
- Add ginger, garlic, and cayenne pepper; cook and stir for 15 seconds.
- Add green onions and chopped mushrooms; cook and stir for 30 seconds.
- Stir cornstarch mixture and add to skillet; cook and stir until boiling.
- Add tofu cubes, pea pods, and sesame oil.

- Cook, stirring gently, for 2 to 3 minutes or until heated through.
- Serve with hot cooked rice and sprinkle with sesame seeds.

Made in United States
Troutdale, OR
11/25/2023